AF541222

Anaesthetic Cocktails for Balanced Anaesthesia A Guide for Small Animal Practitioners

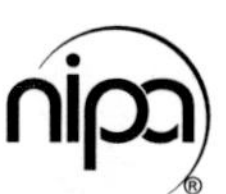

NIPA® GENX ELECTRONIC RESOURCES & SOLUTIONS P. LTD.
New Delhi-110 034

Anaesthetic Cocktails for Balanced Anaesthesia A Guide for Small Animal Practitioners

Sooryadas Surendran
MVSc (Vet. Surgery), PG Dip (Small Animal Theriogenology)
Fellow Vet. Minimal Access Surgery, PhD (Vet. Surgery)
Former Associate Professor & Head (Vet. Surgery & Radiology)
College of Veterinary & Animal Sciences
Kerala Veterinary & Animal Sciences University
Pookode, Wayanad, Kerala.
Chief Surgeon, Charis Veterinary Clinic, Kingdom of Bahrain
Professor and Program Director, Charis Vets Educational, Bahrain

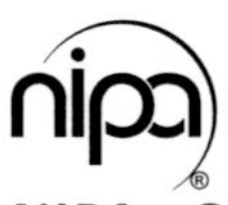

NIPA® GENX ELECTRONIC RESOURCES & SOLUTIONS P. LTD.
New Delhi-110 034

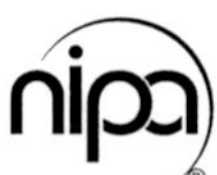

NIPA® GENX ELECTRONIC
RESOURCES & SOLUTIONS P. LTD.
101,103, Vikas Surya Plaza, CU Block
L.S.C.Market, Pitam Pura, New Delhi-110 034
Ph : +91 11 4386 0225, 9717133558, 9540816132
E-mail: newindiapublishingagency@gmail.com
Website: www.nipareources.com

© 2025, Publisher

Print ISBN: 978-93-7219-194-3

ebook ISBN: 978-93-7219-788-4

All rights reserved. No part of this publication may be reproduced, stored in a retrieval system or transmitted in any form or by any means, including electronic, mechanical, photocopying recording or otherwise without the prior written permission of the publisher or the copyright holder.

This book contains information obtained from authentic and highly reliable sources. Reasonable efforts have been made to publish reliable data and information, but the author/s, editor/s and publisher cannot assume responsibility for the validity, accuracy or completeness of all materials or information published herein or the consequences of their use. The work is published with the understanding that the publisher and author/s are not attempting to render any professional services. The author/s, editor/s and publisher have attempted to trace and acknowledge the copyright holders of all material reproduced in this publication and apologize to copyright holders if permission and/or acknowledgements to publish in this form have not been taken. If any copyrighted material has not been acknowledged, please write to us and let us know so that we may rectify the error, in subsequent reprints.

Trademark Notice: NIPA®, the NIPA® logos and their presentations (the way they are written/presented) in this book are the trademarks of the publisher and hence may not be used without written permission, if copied or used without authorization, the infringer will be prosecuted as per law.

NIPA® also publishes books in a variety of electronic formats. Some content that appears in print may not be available in electronic books, and vice versa

Composed and Designed by NIPA®.

Dedication

To my esteemed teachers, who revealed me the subtle art and science of anaesthesia; my speechless patients, whose responses under its influence have taught me more than words ever could; and the two incredible women in my life, whose quiet strength, love, and unwavering support inspired this book.

Preface

The landscape of veterinary anaesthesia has undergone a significant transformation in recent years. The traditional approach of relying on a single or dual anaesthetic drug for sedation and general anaesthesia is giving way to a more refined practice—balanced anaesthesia. The concept of balanced anaesthesia revolves around the careful selection and combination of multiple drugs, each contributing its own targeted effect on neuronal pathways. This method offers the advantage of minimizing the risks and side effects of individual drugs while enhancing the desired outcomes, making it a safer and more effective approach for anaesthesia.

While the theory of balanced anaesthesia is gaining global recognition among veterinary anaesthetists, there are practical challenges that hinder its widespread adoption, especially in regions like India. Many veterinary practitioners in India face significant barriers when it comes to implementing this advanced technique. Lack of resources, such as access to veterinary anaesthesiologists, as well as difficulties in managing the pharmacological dosing of multiple anaesthetic agents, create a complex environment for practitioners. The challenge of memorizing the correct doses and calculating injection volumes—particularly when drugs are measured in different units—further complicates the process. Additionally, the frequent need to open multiple ampoules for each surgery leads to wastage of valuable anaesthetic agents, time, and resources. This often forces practitioners to revert to familiar but suboptimal anaesthetic protocols, relying on just one or two drugs for all procedures, which can increase the risk of adverse effects.

The purpose of this book is to address these challenges by offering a practical and accessible guide to balanced anaesthesia for small animal practitioners. Drawing from both evidence-based research and hands-on clinical experience, this guide proposes a simplified yet effective method for creating balanced anaesthetic cocktails—mixtures of multiple drugs formulated to achieve the desired anaesthetic endpoints. These cocktails are designed to be pharmacologically compatible, easy to administer, and flexible enough to accommodate variations in drug availability across regions.

Each chapter presents a range of anaesthetic cocktail formulations, designed to achieve key behavioural endpoints such as anti-nociception, amnesia, muscle relaxation, and loss of consciousness. The use of lower doses of individual drugs, combined in a balanced manner, reduces the likelihood of side effects and enhances the overall safety of the procedure. Furthermore, the simplified approach of calculating the volume per kilogram body weight enables practitioners to easily determine the correct dose for each animal, eliminating the need for complex calculations.

By offering a more efficient and cost-effective solution, this book aims to equip veterinary practitioners with the tools they need to implement balanced anaesthesia with confidence. It provides a variety of anaesthetic cocktail options that can be tailored to suit the availability of drugs, the type of surgery, and the needs of the animal. Ultimately, this guide is an effort to make balanced anaesthesia more accessible and practical, helping practitioners to provide safer and more effective care for their small animal patients.

Sooryadas S.

Contents

1

Introduction

The yesteryear concept of employing one or two acclaimed anaesthetic drugs to produce sedation and general anaesthesia is now switching over to the era of balanced sedation and balanced anaesthesia. The theory of balanced anaesthesia entails achieving the state of general anaesthesia with the proportionate administration of a mixture of small amounts of several neuronal depressant drugs which summates the advantages of the individual drugs but not their disadvantages (Bettschart-Wolfensberger and Larenza, 2007). Knowledge about balanced anesthesia and targeted effects of drugs on neuronal pathways has started to influence veterinary anaesthetists worldwide. But there are many constraints for a vast majority of veterinary practitioners in India to follow this emerging modality of anaesthetic practice. It is almost impractical for most of them to get the assistance of a veterinary anaesthesiologist every time. So they experience complexities to deal with the pharmacological dosing of multiple component drugs of balanced anaesthetic protocols. Memorising the doses and calculating the volume of injection of multiple component drugs where the doses of some drugs has to be calculated in milligram per kilogram body weight while others have to be calculated in microgram per kilogram body weight becomes a cumbersome task for the practitioner. Moreover, many of these anaesthetic drugs are available in ampoules, and hence multiple ampoules have to be broken for every single surgery; consuming a lot of time. Wastage of the leftover anaesthetic in opened ampoules is another concern. Unavailability of some drugs at some areas is another issue the practitioner faces. These challenges constrain the practitioner from practicing balanced anaesthesia and most of them lean on the verily familiar conventional anaesthetic protocol, based exclusively on one or two frequently used drugs, for almost all the surgical procedures of varying depth. Since only one or two anaesthetic drugs are involved in the protocol, the drugs have to be used at its upper limit of pharmacological doses to achieve the desired endpoints of anaesthesia. This will increase the probable risk of undesired side effects of these drugs.

The challenges that restrict our practitioners from advancing beyond the era of sole reliance on one or two drugs for producing the state of anaesthesia has to be addressed and measures to resolve these issues have to be evolved to promote and equip our veterinary practitioners to practice the safer technique of balanced anaesthesia. Encompassing these objectives, and based on evidence and experience, this book proposes an easy to manoeuver technique of achieving the state of balanced anaesthesia. The technique entails combining different anaesthetic drugs, each with targeted action, at balanced proportion to make an "anaesthetic cocktail" formulation which meets desired behavioural endpoints of anaesthesia. The combinations are physically as well as pharmacologically compatible.

Based on the author's observations from various studies of balanced anaesthesia and clinical practice experience of the same, the chapters places on record various balanced sedative and anaesthetic cocktail preparations useful for a veterinary practitioner. The chapters also provide a supporting brief review of different balanced sedative and anaesthetic drug combinations for dogs and cats.

The classic behavioral endpoints of neurolept anaesthesia/analgesia and general anesthesia like anti nociception, amnesia, loss of consciousness and muscle relaxation are achieved with the small amounts of the individual drugs in the balanced anaesthetic cocktails. The summated effects of multiple anesthetic drugs with targeted endpoint effect will help to achieve more of the desired effects than if the drugs were administered alone, and thereby enable the anesthetist to use each of the drugs at a lower range of its pharmacological dose, reducing the likelihood of undesired after-effects. Practitioners can conveniently use each cocktail as a single entity while achieving the desired behavioral endpoints of all its component drugs. Dosing of the cocktail anesthetic solution is formulated as volume per kilogram body weight regime. Now the practitioner can easily calculate the volume of cocktail anesthetic solution to be administered based on the body weight of the animal. This will relieve the practitioner from deriving the volume of injection of multiple anesthetic drugs from their intricate doses and presentations, for each and every surgical procedure. Administration of calculated volume of the anaesthetic cocktail will provide the state of balanced general anesthesia as all its component drugs maintain its property to achieve the desired individual components of anesthesia. Considering the principle of balanced anesthesia, that the summated effects of component drugs will help to achieve more of the desired effect, the cocktails are formulated in a manner that the concentration of each anesthetic drug in every combination is adjusted to fall in the lower range of its pharmacological dose to achieve the desired effect when administered as per the recommended volume per kilogram regime.

Understanding and addressing the constraints of our veterinary practitioners in India, an honest effort is made to formulate multiple anesthetic cocktails for small animals. Even if some drugs are not available in some areas, practitioners have open options to purchase and prepare different anesthetic cocktail combinations depending upon the availability of component drugs. A single cocktail can be used for multiple surgeries. The inconvenience of breaking multiple ampoules and loading the drugs in multiple syringes for every surgery can be avoided by the onetime preparation of the estimated volume of anesthetic cocktail. Wastage of unused leftover drug in broken ampoules can be limited through this and complete utilization of valuable anesthetic can be ensured. This will conserve the money, energy and time of the practitioner.

Reference

Bettschart-Wolfensberger, R. and Larenza, M.P., 2007. Balanced anesthesia in the equine. Clin. Tech. in Equine Pract., 6(2): 104- 110.

2

Sedative Cocktails

The drug conventionally used for sedation is xylazine, which is an alpha-2 agonist (Dugdale, 2010; Rankin, 2015). Dexmedetomidine is the latest drug of the same class used for sedation, and is more specific to alpha2 receptors than xylazine (Ishyama *et al*., 1995). Doses of 1-2 mg per kg body weight of xylazine (Hall and Clarke, 2001) and upto 20 mcg per kg body weight of dexmedetomidine (Ko, 2013) are required for sedation when used alone (Hall and Clarke, 2001; Rankin, 2015). Similar degrees of sedation could still be achieved at lower doses of xylazine (0.2 to 0.4 mg per kg body weight) and dexmedetomidine (2.5 to 5 mcg per kg) if administered in combination with any opioid drug like hydromorphone / oxymorphone / fentanyl / buprenorphine / butorphanol / nalbuphine / tramadol at their usual doses (Hunt *et al.,* 2013).

Another drug - acepromazine, which is a phenothiazine tranquiliser, is used at its doses of 0.01 to 0.05 mg/kg combined with an opioid for achieving sedation (Smith *et al*., 2001; Dugdale, 2020; Ko, 2013). Combination of an opioid with either a phenothiazine tranquiliser or an alpha2 agonist sedative drug provides neurolept anaesthesia/analgesia (Dugdale, 2020; Rankin, 2015). An anticholinergic drug - glycopyrrolate is administered in combination with acepromazine and opioid to prevent bradycardia (Dyson and James-Davies, 1999). Anticholinergics are generally not recommended with sedative cocktails containing dexmedetomidine, but preferred with sedative cocktails containing xylazine (Congdon *et al.,* 2011; Billah *et al*., 2017). If sedation is to be achieved with acepromazine alone, higher doses need to be administered where there will be an increase in its dose dependent side effects, and hence not preferred (Simon and Steagall, 2020).

Benzodiazepines are another class of sedative drugs, which generally doesn't provide predictable sedation in animals. Paradoxical excitement is caused in healthy adults when these drugs are used alone (Herron *et al*., 2008). Predictable sedation is achieved when these drugs are administered in combination with any opioids (KuKanich and Wiese, 2015). Also, benzodiazepines can be combined with an alpha2-opioid combination to enhance the overall sedation (Maze *et al*., 1992).

Various balanced sedative cocktails prepared with the drugs available for a veterinary practitioner in India, are presented. The balanced sedative cocktails are prepared with either

1) A phenothiazine tranquiliser (acepromazine) and an opioid (buprenorphine/ butorphanol), OR

2) An alpha-2 agonist drug (xylazine/dexmedetomidine) with an opioid (buprenorphine/butorphanol/tramadol/nalbuphine) and a benzodiazepine (midazolam).

Thus, all the cocktails provide neuroleptic-analgesia along with sedation (Hall and Clarke, 2001; Dugdale, 2010). The volume dose of all the balanced sedative cocktail solutions mentioned below is tailored to 0.1 - 0.2 ml per kilogram body weight for dogs and cats, so that the animal receives each individual drug in the combination at their respective recommended doses when administered so. Cats with unruly temperament would require higher doses of the individual drugs and hence 0.4 ml per kilogram body weight is to be administered to achieve similar degrees of sedation. Since these preparations contain either a phenothiazine tranquiliser or an alpha-2 agonist with a benzodiazapine, it is advised that they are prepared in amber-coloured bottles.

Sedative cocktails containing a phenothiazine tranquiliser along with an opioid and an anticholinergic

The combinations provide analgesia as well as sedation, more than when the individual drugs are used alone (Ralh and Mohindroo, 2010; Barvalia *et al*., 2013). Also, the incidence of adverse effects is reduced (Short *et al.,* 1997). Combining glycopyrrolate - an anticholinergic, will prevent bradycardia and maintain the heart rate (Dyson and James-Davies, 1999).

The combinations can be given intramuscular as well as intravenous. Intravenous administration can be done for animals permitting the same, where the lower volume dose should be chosen. Intramuscular route can be chosen for those animals that do not permit intravenous administration, where the higher volume dose should be chosen.

1. Buprenorphine/Butorphanol-Acepromazine-Glycopyrrolate (BAG)

Preparation when buprenorphine is used.......

Drugs (presentation)	Vol. to be taken	Total mg/mcg of the drug	Conc. of individual drugs in the sedative cocktail solution
Buprenorphine (0.3 mg/ml)	3.4 ml	1.02 mg	Buprenorphine = 0.051 mg/ml
Acepromazine (10 mg/ml)	0.5 ml	5.0 mg	Acepromazine = 0.25 mg/ml
Glycopyrrolate (0.2 mg/ml)	5.0 ml	1.0 mg	Glycopyrrolate = 0.05 mg/ml
Dist. water for Inj.	11.1 ml	....	....
TOTAL	20 ml	....	....

Dose = @ 0.1 to 0.2 ml/kg IV/IM (1 to 2 ml per 10 kg IV/IM) for dogs and cats

Administering this volume provides
Buprenorphine @ 0.005-0.01 mg/kg
Acepromazine @ 0.025-0.05 mg/kg
Glycopyrrolate @ 0.005-0.01 mg/kg

The cost of the preparation would be approximately Rs. 13 per ml as per the MRP of each of the drugs.

Preparation when butorphanol is used.......

Drugs (presentation)	Vol. to be taken	Total mg/mcg of the drug	Conc. of individual drugs in the sedative cocktail solution
Butorphanol (2 mg/ml)	14.6 ml	29.2 mg	Butorphanol = 1.46 mg/ml
Acepromazine (10 mg/ml)	0.4 ml	4.0 mg	Acepromazine = 0.2 mg/ml
Glycopyrrolate (0.2 mg/ml)	5.0 ml	1.0 mg	Glycopyrrolate = 0.05 mg/ml
TOTAL	20 ml	....	....
Dose = @ 0.1 to 0.2 ml/kg IV/IM (1 to 2 ml per 10 kg IV/IM) for dogs and cats			
			Administering this volume provides Butorphanol @ 0.146-0.292 mg/kg Acepromazine @ 0.02-0.04 mg/kg Glycopyrrolate @ 0.005-0.01 mg/kg

The cost of the preparation would be approximately Rs. 58 per ml as per the MRP of each of the drugs.

The above combinations provide mild to moderate sedation along with mild to moderate analgesia. Degree of sedation depends on the route of administration, temperament of the patient, and also the health status of the animal. Generally, the buprenorphine-containing combination provides mild sedation, while that containing butorphanol provides moderate sedation (Bhalla *et al.,* 2017). Both combinations should be used with caution in Boxers, giant breeds of dogs, and severely hypovolaemic patients (Pawson, 2008).

These combinations can be used for mild to moderate sedation and analgesia, permitting physical examinations and radiographic positioning which involve only mild to moderate degree of pain. Also, this can be used as a balanced pre-anaesthetic medication to produce mild to moderate degree of sedation and analgesia which could then be followed by injectable agents for induction of general anaesthesia.

If induction of general anaesthesia is to be proceeded with an intravenous anaesthetic induction agent like propofol or thiopentone, following administration of the above combination, the dose(s) of the induction drug(s) should be reduced depending on the depth of sedation achieved with the above combination, or the anesthetic induction drug should be administered "to effect" (Ralh and Monindroo, 2010; Shah *et al.,* 2011).

Sedative cocktails containing an alpha-2 agonist along with an opioid and a benzodiazepine

An opioid along with a benzodiazepine will help reduce the dose of an alpha-2 agonist like xylazine or dexmedetomidine used in combination with them to effect sedation (Dugdale, 2010; Ko, 2013). The opioid can be any of those available for veterinary practice in India like butorphanol or buprenorphine or tramadol or nalbuphine. The benzodiazepine preferred in all the preparations is midazolam because it is water-soluble, will not precipitate when mixed with any of the other drugs mentioned above, can be given intravenously as well as intramuscular, and absorption from intramuscular injection sites is better than its counterpart - diazepam (Hung *et al.*, 1996).

1. Xylazine-Butorphanol / Buprenorphine-Midazolam (XBM)

Preparation when butorphanol is used .....

Drugs (presentation)	Vol. to be taken	Total mg/mcg of the drug	Conc. of individual drugs in the sedative cocktail solution
Xylazine (20 mg/ml)	2 ml	40 mg	Xylazine = 2 mg/ml
Butorphanol (2 mg/ml)	10 ml	20 mg	Butorphanol = 1 mg/ml
Midazolam (5mg/ml)	5 ml	25 mg	Midazolam = 1.25 mg/ml
Dist. Water for Inj.	3 ml	....	....
Total	20 ml	....	....

Dose = 0.1 - 0.2 ml/kg IM (1 - 2 ml/10 kg) for dogs and cats

Administering this volume provides
Xylazine @ 0.2 - 0.4 mg/kg
Butorphanol @ 0.1 - 0.2 mg/kg
Midazolam @ 0.125 - 0.25 mg/kg

The cost of the preparation would be approximately Rs. 40 per ml as per the MRP of each of the drugs.

Preparation when buprenorphine is used ....

Drugs (presentation)	Vol. to be taken	Total mg/mcg of the drug	Conc. of individual drugs in the sedative cocktail solution
Xylazine (20 mg/ml)	2 ml	40 mg	Xylazine = 2 mg/ml
Buprenorphine (0.3 mg/ml)	3.4 ml	1.02 mg	Buprenorphine = 0.051 mg/ml
Midazolam (5mg/ml)	5 ml	25 mg	Midazolam = 1.25 mg/ml
Dist. Water for Inj.	9.6 ml	....	....
TOTAL	20 ml	....	....

Dose = 0.1 - 0.2 ml/kg IM (1 - 2 ml/10 kg) for dogs and cats

Administering this volume provides
Xylazine @ 0.2 - 0.4 mg/kg
Buprenorphine @ 0.005 - 0.01 mg/kg
Midazolam @ 0.125 - 0.25 mg/kg

The cost of the preparation would be approximately Rs. 12 per ml as per the MRP of each of the drugs.

2. Xylazine-Nalbuphine-Midazolam (XNM)

The butorphanol in the XBM cocktail is replaced by 10 mg/ml presentation of nalbuphine (Pallasch and Gill, 1985; Lester *et al.,* 2003) at the same volume of 10 ml as that of butorphanol, for preparation of this combination. When replaced, nalbuphine will be 5 mg/ml in the preparation, and when administered at the said volume, will provide nalbuphine @ 0.5 - 1 mg/kg (Ko, 2013).

Drugs (presentation)	Vol. to be taken	Total mg/mcg of the drug	Conc. of individual drugs in the sedative cocktail solution
Xylazine (20 mg/ml)	2 ml	40 mg	Xylazine = 2 mg/ml
Nalbuphine (10 mg/ml)	10 ml	100 mg	Nalbuphine = 5 mg/ml
Midazolam (5mg/ml)	5 ml	25 mg	Midazolam = 1.25 mg/ml
Dist. Water for Inj.	3 ml	....	....
Total	20 ml	....	....
Dose = 0.1 - 0.2 ml/kg IM (1 - 2 ml/10 kg) for dogs and cats			
			Administering this volume provides Xylazine @ 0.2 - 0.4 mg/kg Nalbuphine @ 0.5 - 1.0 mg/kg Midazolam @ 0.125 - 0.25 mg/kg

The cost of the preparation would be approximately Rs.31 per ml as per the MRP of each of the drugs.

3. Xylazine-Tramadol-Midazolam (XTraM)

Butorphanol in the XBM cocktail is replaced by 50 mg/ml presentation of tramadol at the same volume of 10 ml as that of butorphanol, for preparation of this combination. When replaced, tramadol will be 25 mg/ml in the preparation, and when administered at the said volume, will provide tramadol @ 2.5 - 5 mg/kg body weight (Dugdale, 2010).

Drugs (presentation)	Vol. to be taken	Total mg/mcg of the drug	Conc. of individual drugs in the sedative cocktail solution
Xylazine (20 mg/ml)	2 ml	40 mg	Xylazine = 2 mg/ml
Tramadol (50 mg/ml)	10 ml	500 mg	Tramadol = 25 mg/ml
Midazolam (5mg/ml)	5 ml	25 mg	Midazolam = 1.25 mg/ml
Dist. Water for Inj.	3 ml	....	....
TOTAL	20 ml	....	....
Dose = 0.1 - 0.2 ml/kg IM (1 - 2 ml/10 kg) for dogs and cats			
			Administering this volume provides Xylazine @ 0.2 - 0.4 mg/kg Tramadol @ 2.5 - 5.0 mg/kg Midazolam @ 0.125 - 0.25 mg/kg

The cost of the preparation would be approximately Rs.12 per ml as per the MRP of each of the drugs.

2. Dexmedetomidine-Butorphanol/Buprenorphine-Midazolam (DBM)

Preparation when butorphanol is used

Drugs (presentation)	Vol. to be taken	Total mg/mcg of the drug	Conc. of individual drugs in the sedative cocktail solution
Dexmedetomidine (100 mcg/ml)	5 ml	500 mcg	Dexmedetomidine = 25 mcg/ml
Butorphanol (2 mg/ml)	10 ml	20 mg	Butorphanol = 1 mg/ml
Midazolam (5mg/ml)	5 ml	25 mg	Midazolam = 1.25 mg/ml
Dist. water for Inj.	....	....	....
Total	20 ml	....	....
Dose = 0.1 - 0.2 ml/kg IM (1 - 2 ml/10 kg IM) for dogs and cats			
			Administering this volume provides Dexmedetomidine @ 2.5 - 5 mcg/kg, Butorphanol @ 0.1 - 0.2 mg/kg Midazolam @ 0.125 - 0.25 mg/kg

The cost of the preparation would be approximately Rs. 168 per ml as per the MRP of each of the drugs..

Preparation when buprenorphine is used

Drugs (presentation)	Vol. to be taken	Total mg/mcg of the drug	Conc. of individual drugs in the sedative cocktail solution
Dexmedetomidine (100 mcg/ml)	5 ml	500 mcg	Dexmedetomidine = 25 mcg/ml
Buprenorphine (0.3 mg/ml)	3.4 ml	1.02 mg	Buprenorphine = 0.051 mg/ml
Midazolam (5mg/ml)	5 ml	25 mg	Midazolam = 1.25 mg/ml
Dist. water for Inj.	6.6 ml	....	....
TOTAL	20 ml	....	....
Dose = 0.1 - 0.2 ml/kg IM (1 - 2 ml/10 kg IM) for dogs and cats			
			Administering this volume provides Dexmedetomidine @ 2.5 - 5 mcg/kg, Buprenorphine @ 0.005 - 0.01 mg/kg Midazolam @ 0.125 - 0.25 mg/kg

The cost of the preparation would be approximately Rs. 139 per ml as per the MRP of each of the drugs.

All of the above combinations can be administered intramuscular as well as intravenous. Intramuscular administration is preferred.

Sedative cocktails containing buprenorphine/tramadol/nalbuphine provide only mild to moderate sedation which could be used for physical examinations and radiographic positioning which involve only mild to moderate degree of pain. If moderate to profound sedation is desired, combinations containing butorphanol shall be used, which permits procedures involving moderate degree of pain. For procedures involving severe degree of pain, ketamine at its analgesic dose should be either included with the combination or separately administered IV following sedation (Slingsby and Pearson, 2000; Brown and Tucker, 2020).

The degree of sedation achieved with the above sedative cocktails depends on the temperament of the animal and the dose administered (Vesce, 2015; Filippi, 2015). If the animal is disturbed following the administration of the sedative cocktails, the level of sedation may not be achieved at its desired depth (Ilkkaya *et al.*, 2014; Albright *et al.,* 2017). Cats, following administration of the sedative cocktails, should be kept confined in its carrier basket away from light. Else, the expected level of sedation would not be achieved (Robertson *et al.,* 2018).

Since the sedation achieved with cocktails containing xylazine/ dexmedetomidine with butorphanol is most often profound (Sharma *et al.*, 2014; Sahoo *et al.,* 2018), the dose(s) of intravenous anaesthetic induction drugs like propofol and thiopentone should be greatly reduced (75% or more reduced depending on the depth of sedation) or should be diluted and administered "titrated to effect" (Kumari *et al.,* 2018) for induction of general anaesthesia, if needed.

The above sedative cocktails can be administered intravenously for those animals permitting the same, but the lower volume dose should be chosen. Quick and profound sedation can happen with intravenous administration, and hence, the patient's cardiopulmonary parameters should be very closely monitored when combinations are administered intravenously (Sheahan and Mathews, 2014). Intravenous administration may be practiced by those well equipped with anaesthetic monitoring facilities and capable of managing emergency situations that may arise if any.

References

Albright, J.D., Seddighi, R.M., Zenithson, N.G., Sun, X. and Rezac, D.J. 2017. Effect of environmental noise and music on dexmedetomidine-induced sedation in dogs. PeerJ [online] Available: https://peerj.com/articles/3659/ published July 31, 2017. doi: 10.7717/peerj.3659.

Barvalia, D.R., Ranpariya, J.J., Padaliya, N.R. and Javia, C.B. 2013. Safety and efficacy of butorphanol-acepromazine-glycopyrrolate as premedicant combination to midazolam-ketamine induction and isoflurane maintenance in canine orthopaedic surgery. Indian J. Field Vet. 9(1): 30-34.

Bhalla, R.J., Trimble, T.A., Leece, E.A. and Vettorato, E. 2017. Comparison of intramuscular butorphanol and buprenorphine combined with dexmedetomidine for sedation in cats. J. Feline. Med. Surg. 20(4): 325–331.

Billah, A. M., Sultana, S., Hossain, M. A., Hashim, M. A., Begum, T., Rahman, B. and Rashid, M. 2017. Evaluation of different premedicants in canine anaesthesia. Res. Agri. Livestock Fish. 4(3): 209.

Brown, K. and Tucker, C. 2020. Ketamine for acute pain management and sedation. Crit. Care Nurse. 40(5): 26-32.

Congdon, J. M., Marquez, M., Niyom, S., and Boscan, P. 2011. Evaluation of the sedative and cardiovascular effects of intramuscular administration of dexmedetomidine with and without concurrent atropine administration in dogs. J. Am. Vet. Med. Ass. 239(1): 81–89.

Dugdale, A. 2010. Veterinary Anaesthesia Principles to Practice, 2nd Ed., Wiley Blackwell Publishing, U.S.A., p. 30-42.

Dugdale, A.H.A., Beaumont, G., Bradbrook, C. and Gurney, M. 2020. Sedation and Premedication Small Animals In: Veterinary Anaesthesia Principles to Practice (2nd ed.). Wiley Blackwell Publishing, U.S.A. pp. 55-76.

Dyson, D.H. and James-Davies, R. 1999. Dose, effect and benefits of glycopyrrolate in the treatment of bradycardia in anesthetized dogs. Can. Vet. J. 40(5): 327–331.

Filippi, C. 2015. Sedation of anxious, fearful and/or aggressive dogs [abstract]. Compendium, Proceedings of the 1st International Conference on One Anaesthesia: Focus on Sedation. 25&26 May 2015. In: Minerva Anestesiologica, Official Journal of Italian Society of Anaesthesiology, Analgesia, Resuscitation and Intensive Care. 81(1-7): 7-8.

Hall, L.W., Clarke, K.W. and Trim, C.M. 2001. Principles of sedation, analgesia and premedication In: Veterinary Anaesthesia. 10th Ed. London, Saunders. p. 101.

Herron, M. E., Shofer, F. S., and Reisner, I. R. 2008. Retrospective evaluation of the effects of diazepam in dogs with anxiety-related behavior problems. J. Am. Vet. Med. Ass. 233(9): 1420–1424.

Hung, O. R., Dyck, J. B., Varvel, J., Shafer, S. L., and Stanski, D. R. 1996. Comparative absorption kinetics of intramuscular midazolam and diazepam. Can. J. Anaesth. 43(5), 450–455.

Hunt, J.R., Grint, N.J., Taylor, P.M. and Murrell, J.C. 2013 Sedative and analgesic effects of buprenorphine, combined with either acepromazine or dexmedetomidine, for premedication prior to elective surgery in cats and dogs. Vet. Anaesth. Analg.40: 297–307.

Ilkkaya, N. K., Ustun, F. E., Sener, E. B., Kaya, C., Ustun, Y. B., Koksal, E. and Ozkan, F. 2014. The Effects of Music, White Noise, and Ambient Noise on Sedation and Anxiety in Patients Under Spinal Anesthesia During Surgery. J. Peri Anesthesia Nurs.,29(5): 418–426.

Ishiyama, T., Dohi, S., Iida, H., Watanabe, Y. and Shimonaka, H. 1995. Mechanisms of dexmedetomidine-induced cerebrovascular effects in canine in vivo experiments. Anesth. Analg. 81(6), 1208–1215.

Ko, J.C. 2013. Preanesthetic medication: drugs and dosages. In: Small animal anaesthesia and pain management - A color handbook, Mansion Publishing Ltd.pp. 59-85.

Kumari, A., Singh, A., Vidhan, J. and Gupta, R. 2018. The Sedative and Propofol-Sparing Effect of Dexmedetomidine and Midazolam as Premedicants in Minor Gynecological Day Care Surgeries: A Randomized Placebo-Controlled Study. Anesthesia Essays Res. 12(2): 423-427.

KuKanich, B. and Wiese, J.A., 2015. Opioids. In: Lumb and Jones Veterinary Anaesthesia and Analgesia, 5th Ed., Grimm, K.A., Lamont, L.A., Tranquilli, W.J., Greene, S.A. and Roberston, S.A. Wiley Blackwell Publishing, U.S.A. p. 212.

Lester, P.A., Gaynor, J.S., Hellyer, P.W., Mama, K.R. and Wagner, A.E. 2003. The Sedative and Behavioral Effects of Nalbuphine in Dogs. Contemp. Topics Am. Ass. Lab. Anim. Sci.42(4): 27-31.

Maze, M., Salonen, M. and Reid, K., 1992. Synergistic Interaction Between α2-Adrenergic Agonists and Benzodiazepines in Rats. Anesthesiology. 76(6):1004–1011.

Pallasch, T. J., and Gill, C. J. 1985. Butorphanol and nalbuphine: A pharmacologic comparison. Oral Surg., Oral Med., Oral Path.59(1): 15–20.

Pawson P. 2008. Sedatives. In: Maddison, J.E., Page, S.P., and Church, D. Small Animal Clinical Pharmacology, 2nd Ed., Elsevier, Philadelphia., p. 113-125.

Ralh, P. and Mohindroo, J. 2010. Evaluation of butorphanol-acepromazine-glycopyrrolate and butorphanol-midazolam-glycopyrrolate as preanaesthetic to thiopentoneanaesthesia in dogs. Indian. J. Vet. Surg. 31(2): 123-126.

Rankin, D.C. 2015. Sedatives and Tranquilizers. In: Lumb and Jones Veterinary Anaesthesia and Analgesia, 5th Ed., Grimm, K.A., Lamont, L.A., Tranquilli, W.J., Greene, S.A. and Robertson, S.A. Wiley Blackwell Publishing, U.S.A., p. 196-199.

Robertson, S. A., Gogolski, S. M., Pascoe, P., Shafford, H. L., Sager, J., and Griffenhagen, G. M. 2018. AAFP Feline Anesthesia Guidelines. J. Feline Med. Surg.20(7): 602–634.

Sahoo, M., Nath, I., Nayak, S., Kundu, A.K., Panda, S.K. and Patra, B. 2018. Comparison of sedative effect of Dexmedetomidine/ Xylazine in combination with Butorphanol-Midazolam as preanaesthetic to Ketamine anaesthesia for ovariohysterectomy in dogs. Exploratory Anim. Med. Res. 8(1) 79-84.

Shah, N.K., Harris, M., Govindugari, K., Rangaswamy, H.B. and Jeon, H. 2011. Effect of propofol titration v/s bolus during induction of anesthesia on hemodynamics and bispectral index. Middle East J. Anaesth. 21(2):275-81.

Sharma, R., Kumar, A., Kumar, A., Sharma, S.K., Sharma, A. and Tewari, N. 2014. Comparison of xylazine and dexmedetomidine as a premedicant for general anaesthesia in dogs. Indian. J. Anim. Sci. 84(1): 8-12.

Sheahan, C. G. and Mathews, D. M. 2014. Monitoring and delivery of sedation. Brit. J. Anaesth. 113(2): 37-47.

Short, C. E., Bufalari, A., Miller, S. M., and Giannoni, G. 1997. The use of propofol for induction of anaesthesia in dogs premedicated with acepromazine, butorphanol and acepromazine-butorphanol. N. Z. Vet. J. 45(4), 129–134.

Simon, B. T. and Steagall, P. V. 2020. Feline procedural sedation and analgesia: When, why and how. J. Feline Med. Surg. 22(11): 1029–1045.

Slingsby, L. and Pearson., A.W. 2000. The post-operative analgesic effects of ketamine after canine ovariohysterectomy—a comparison between pre- or post-operative administration. Res. Vet. Sci. 69(2), 147–152.

Smith, L. J., Yu, J.A., Bjorling, D. E., and Waller, K. 2001. Effects of hydromorphone or oxymorphone, with or without acepromazine, on preanesthetic sedation, physiologic values, and histamine release in dogs. J. Am. Vet. Med. Ass. 218(7): 1101–1105.

Vesce, G. 2015. Clinical implications of sedation in animals [abstract]. Compendium, Proceedings of the 1st International Conference on One Anaesthesia: Focus on Sedation. 25&26 May 2015. In: Minerva Anestesiologica, Official Journal of Italian Society of Anaesthesiology, Analgesia, Resuscitation and Intensive Care. 81(1-7): 16-17.

3

Induction Cocktails

Ketamine and Propofol - "Ketofol"

"Ketofol" is a 1:1 (w:w) combination of ketamine and propofol (Taboada and Leece, 2014; Thejasree *et al.*, 2018). The advantages of using both ketamine and propofol in combination (Ketofol) include analgesia, rapid recovery, preservation of airways and maintenance of spontaneous respiration and haemodynamic stability (Saeed, 2011). The admixture has benefits of both drugs, while reducing the side effects of the individual drugs when administered alone (Amornyotin, 2014; Lee and Lee, 2016; Mirfazaelian *et al.*, 2016). Propofol-induced respiratory depression is less with the admixture, while analgesia and cardiorespiratory functions are good due to ketamine (Amornyotin, 2014; Mirfazaelian *et al.*, 2016). Since the adverse effects are dose dependent, the combination helps reduce the dose of the individual drug needed to cause the desired anaesthetic effects.

Preparation of Ketofol

Drugs (presentation)	Vol. to be taken	Total mg/mcg of the drug	Conc. of individual drugs in the induction cocktail solution
Ketamine (50 mg/ml)	2 ml	100 mg	Ketamine = 5 mg/ml
Propofol (10 mg/ml)	10 ml	100 mg	Propofol = 5 mg/ml
Normal saline/Dist. water	8 ml	....	....
Total	20 ml	....	Ketofol = 10 mg/ml

Dose = @ 0.2-0.4 ml/kg (1-2 ml/5 kg IV) for dogs and cats (Adjustment of the dose shall be needed based on the depth of sedation achieved with the sedative cocktail)

Administering this volume provides
Ketamine @ 1-2 mg/kg
Propofol @ 1-2 mg/kg

The cost of the preparation would be approximately Rs. 5 per ml as per the MRP of each of the drugs.

This combination of ketamine and propofol can be used to induce anaesthesia following sedation with any of the previously mentioned balanced sedative cocktails. Induction should be "titrated to effect" based on the depth of sedation achieved from the administration of the balanced sedative cocktails.

Thiopentone and Propofol - "Thio-propofol"

Thio-propofol is a 1:1 vol:vol mixture of 2.5% thiopentone and 1% propofol (Ko *et al.*, 1999; Evans *et al.*, 2002; Larisa *et al.*, 2008). Since the mechanisms of action of propofol and thiopentone are similar, the mixture provides an additive hypnotic interaction (Vinik *et al.*, 1999) and behaves in-between to that of the individual drugs (Ko *et al.*, 1999). Using this mixture, non-premedicated dogs required a mean 2.7 mg/kg propofol and 6.8 mg/kg thiopentone (Ko *et al.*, 1999) to allow endotracheal intubation. Premedicated dogs required 2.5 to 4 mg/kg propofol and 6.5 to 10 mg/kg thiopentone (Larisa *et al.*, 2008) to allow endotracheal intubation. Respiratory depression happens with administration of the mixture, but is not that severe as with the individual agents. The anaesthetic recovery is almost faster and smoother than that with thiopentone alone (Ko *et al.*, 1999). Since the mixture does not support bacterial growth (Crowther *et al.*, 1996) the preparation can be stored for further use.

Preparation of Thio-propofol

Drugs (presentation)	Vol. to be taken	Total mg/mcg of the drug	Conc. of individual drugs in the induction cocktail solution
2.5% (25 mg/ml) Thiopentone solution (reconstitute 500 mg thiopentone with 20 ml dist water to prepare 2.5% solution)	20 ml	500 mg	Thiopentone = 12.5 mg/ml
1% (10 mg/ml) Propofol	20 ml	200 mg	Propofol = 5 mg/ml
Total	40 ml	....	
Dose =	**For dogs sedated following premedication** Take at 0.1 - 0.2 ml/kg (1-2 ml/10 kg) in a syringe, extend it five times its volume using distilled water, and administer IV "to effect" (Adjustment of the dose shall be needed based on the depth of sedation achieved with the sedative cocktail) Administering this full volume provides Thiopentone @ 1.25 - 2.5 mg/kg Propofol @ 0.5 - 1 mg/kg **For non-premedicated dogs** Take at 0.5 - 0.6 ml/kg (5-6 ml/10 kg) in a syringe, extend it twice to its vol using dist water, and administer IV "to effect". Administering this full volume provides Thiopentone @ 6.25 - 7.5 mg/kg Propofol @ 2.5 - 3 mg/kg		

References

Amornyotin S. 2014. Ketofol: A Combination of Ketamine and Propofol. J Anesth. Crit. Care. 1(5): 00031.

Crowther, J., Hrazdil, J., Jolly, D.T., Galbraith, J.C., Greacen, M. and Grace, M. 1996. Growth of microorganisms in Propofol, Thiopental, and a 1:1 Mixture of Propofol and Thiopental. Anesth. Analg. 82: 475

Evans, A.T., Anderson, L.K. and Hauptman, J. 2002. Echocardiographic evaluation of dogs receiving 1:1 thiopental/propofol in a clinical setting. Proceedings of the American College of Veterinary Anesthesiologists 27th Annual Meeting, Orlando, Florida, 10&11 October 2002 In Meeting Abstracts Veterinary Anaesthesia and Analgesia, 2003, 30:102.

Ko, J.C., Golder, F.J., Mandsager, R.E., Heaton-Jones, T.G. and Mattern, K.L. 1999. Anesthetic and cardiorespiratory effects of a 1:1 mixture of propofol and thiopental sodium in dogs. J. Am. Vet. Med. Assoc.215:1292

Larisa, S., Igna, C. and Sala, A. 2008. Propofol-Thiopental mixture in brachycephalic dogs prepared for myelography. Bulletin UASVM, Vet. Med. 65(2): 212-216

Lee. K. C and Lee. B.C. 2016. Ketofol as a Balanced Anesthetic for Procedural Sedation and Analgesia in the Obese Oral Surgery Patient: a Commentary. Int. J. Dentistry Oral Sci. 03(2), 190-192.

Mirfazaelian, H., Jalili, M., Bahreini, M., Doosti-Irani, A., Masoomi, R. and Arbab, M. 2016. Ketamine-propofol combination (ketofol) vs propofol for procedural sedation and analgesia: systematic review and meta-analysis. Am. J. Emergency Med. 34(3), 558–569.

Saeed, E. 2011. Ketofol Infusion as a procedural sedation and analgesia modality for minor orthopaedic surgeries: evaluation of dose-outcome relation. Ain Shams J. Anaesthesiology. 4(1): 63-74.

Taboada, F.M. and Leece, E.A., 2014. Comparison of propofol with ketofol, a propofol-ketamine admixture for induction of anaesthesia in healthy dogs. Vet. Anaes. Analg., 41(6): 575-582.

Thejasree, P., Veena, P., Dhanalakshmi, N., and Veerabrahmaiah, K. 2018. Evaluation of Propofol and Ketofol Anaesthesia Following Atropine, Diazepam and Fentanyl Premedication in Dogs. Int. J. Curr. Microbiol. App. Sci., 7(11): 3130-3137.

Vinik, H.R., Bradley, E.L. and Kissin, I. 1999, Isoholographic analysis of propofol-thiopental hypnotic interaction in surgical patients. Anesth. analg. 88(3): 667-670.

4

Anaesthetic Cocktails

Combination of an opioid (butorphanol/buprenorphine) and an alpha-2 agonist (xylazine/dexmedetomidine) along with an NMDA antagonist and benzodiazepine (tiletamine-zolazepam or ketamine-midazolam) will make up a balanced anaesthetic cocktail. Examples for balanced anaesthetic cocktails are xylazine/dexmedetomidine-butorphanol-midazolam-ketamine and butorphanol/buprenorphine-tiletamine zolazepam-dexmedetomidine/xylazine (Ko, 2013; Cagle *et al.*, 2017; Sooryadas *et al.*, 2019; Verma *et al.*, 2020). The latter ones are costly due to the tiletamine-zolazepam and dexmedetomidine in them, while the former ones are cost effective alternatives.

Xylazine/Dexmedetomidine-Butorphanol-Midazolam-Ketamine (XBMK/DBMK) Anaesthetic Cocktail

The preparation can be made by drawing 0.1 ml/kg of ketamine (50 mg/ml presentation) along with 0.1 to 0.2 ml/kg of the xylazine-butorphanol-midazolam (XBM) or dexmedetomidine-butorphanol-midazolam (DBM) sedative cocktail in a single syringe. For intravenous administration, 0.1 ml/kg each of ketamine and the sedative cocktail is to be chosen, while for intramuscular administration 0.1 ml/kg of ketamine and 0.2 ml/kg of the sedative cocktail is preferred. The volume of the cocktail that needs to be administered intramuscularly will be larger by 0.1 ml/kg when compared to the tiletamine-zolazepam based anaesthetic cocktails. Anticholinergic premedication is preferred prior to administration of anaesthetic cocktail containing xylazine (Nesgash *et al.*, 2016), particularly if given intravenously. The XBMK/DBMK anaesthetic cocktails will induce anaesthesia in a few minutes, which last for 20 to 40 minutes (Ko, 2013; Verma *et al.*, 2019; Verma *et al.*, 2020). Intravenous administration of the anaesthetic cocktail provides shorter duration of surgical plane of anaesthesia. When administered as said above, the combination provides xylazine @ 0.2 - 0.4 mg/kg or dexmedetomidine @ 2.5 - 5 mcg/kg, butorphanol @ 0.1 - 0.2 mg/kg, midazolam @ 0.125 - 0.25 mg/kg and ketamine @ 5 mg/kg body weight which is as per their recommended doses when given in combination (Verma *et al.*, 2019; Verma *et al.*, 2020).

Preparation of XBMK anaesthetic cocktail .....

Vol of the drugs to be taken in a single syringe for the anaesthetic cocktail		Route	Dose of the individual drugs received when administered
Ketamine (50 mg/ml)	XBM sedative cocktail		
0.1 ml/kg	0.1 ml/kg	IV	Xylazine @ 0.2 mg/kg Butorphanol @ 0.1 mg/kg Midazolam @ 0.125 mg/kg Ketamine @ 5 mg/kg
0.1 ml/kg	0.2 ml/kg	IM	Xylazine @ 0.4 mg/kg Butorphanol @ 0.2 mg/kg Midazolam @ 0.25 mg/kg Ketamine @ 5 mg/kg

Preparation of DBMK anaesthetic cocktail .....

Vol of the drugs to be taken in a single syringe for the anaesthetic cocktail		Route	Dose of the individual drugs received when administered
Ketamine (50 mg/ml)	DBM sedative cocktail		
0.1 ml/kg	0.1 ml/kg	IV	Dexmedetomindine @ 2.5 mcg/kg Butorphanol @ 0.1 mg/kg Midazolam @ 0.125 mg/kg Ketamine @ 5 mg/kg
0.1 ml/kg	0.2 ml/kg	IM	Dexmedetomindine @ 5 mcg/kg Butorphanol @ 0.2 mg/kg Midazolam @ 0.25 mg/kg Ketamine @ 5 mg/kg

Butorphanol/ Buprenorphine - Tiletamine Zolazepam-Dexmedetomidine/ Xylazine (BTDex/BTX)

The tiletamine-zolazepam powder is reconstituted with either butorphanol and dexmedetomidine, or buprenorphine, dexmedetomidine and distilled water to form BTDex. The tiletamine-zolazepam powder can also be reconstituted with butorphanol/buprenorphine, xylazine and distilled water to form BTX anaesthetic cocktail. These anaesthetic cocktails can be used in dogs as well as cats for chemical restraint, premedication and surgery (Ko *et al.*, 2012; Ko, 2013). Following a single intramuscular injection, the BTDex and BTX combinations provide various depths of sedation and even surgical plane of anaesthesia. The same combination can be used both in dogs and cats, at the same dose rates. The combination provides visceral as well as somatic analgesia. Based on evidence (Ko and Berman, 2010; Ko and Krimins, 2013) and clinical experience, the above cocktails can be stored at room temperature upto three months following reconstitution, and it is recommended not to store the mixture in the refrigerator.

2a) Butorphanol/ Buprenorphine - Tiletamine Zolazepam-Dexmedetomidine (BTDex)

Preparation when butorphanol is used.....

Drugs (presentation)	Vol. to be taken	Total mg/mcg of the drug	Conc. of individual drugs in the anaesthetic cocktail solution
Butorphanol (2 mg/ml)	6.25 ml	12.5 mg	Butorphanol = 1 mg/ml
Tiletamine-Zolazepam (ZOLETIL-50) (125 mg Tiletamine & 125 mg Zolazepam)	Powder	250 mg	TiletamineZolazepam = 20 mg/ml (Tiletamine 10 mg/ml & Zolazepam 10 mg/ml)
Dexmedetomidine (100 mcg/ml)	6.25 ml	625 mcg	Dexmedetomidine = 50 mcg/ml
Total	12.50 ml	....	....

The cost of the preparation would be approximately Rs. 449 per ml as per the MRP of each of the drugs.

Preparation when buprenorphine is used.....

Drugs (presentation)	Vol. to be taken	Total mg/mcg of the drug	Conc. of individual drugs in the anaesthetic cocktail solution
Buprenorphine (0.3 mg/ml)	1.25 ml	0.375 mg	Buprenorphine = 0.03 mg/ml
Tiletamine-Zolazepam (ZOLETIL-50) (125 mg Tiletamine & 125 mg Zolazepam)	Powder	250 mg	TiletamineZolazepam = 20 mg/ml (Tiletamine 10 mg/ml & Zolazepam 10 mg/ml)
Dexmedetomidine (100 mcg/ ml)	6.25 ml	625 mcg	Dexmedetomidine = 50 mcg/ml
Dist. water for Inj.	5.0 ml	....	....
Total	12.50 ml	....	....

The cost of the preparation would be approximately Rs. 415 per ml as per the MRP of each of the drugs.

2b) Butorphanol/Buprenorphine-TiletamineZolazepam-Xylazine (BTX)

Preparation when butorphanol is used.....

Drugs (presentation)	Vol. to be taken	Total mg/mcg of the drug	Conc. of individual drugs in the anaesthetic cocktail solution
Butorphanol (2 mg/ml)	6.25 ml	12.5 mg	Butorphanol = 1 mg/ml
Tiletamine-Zolazepam (ZOLETIL-50) (125 mg Tiletamine & 125 mg Zolazepam)	Powder	250 mg	TiletamineZolazepam = 20 mg/ml (Tiletamine 10 mg/ml & Zolazepam 10 mg/ml)
Xylazine (20 mg/ml)	1.25 ml	25 mg	Xylazine = 2 mg/ml
Dist. water for Inj.	5 ml	....	....
Total	12.50 ml	....	....

The cost of the preparation would be approximately Rs. 160 per ml as per the MRP of each of the drugs.

Preparation when buprenorphine is used.....

Drugs (presentation)	Vol. to be taken	Total mg/mcg of the drug	Conc. of individual drugs in the anaesthetic cocktail solution
Buprenorphine (0.3 mg/ml)	1.25 ml	0.375 mg	Buprenorphine = 0.03 mg/ml
Tiletamine-Zolazepam (ZOLETIL-50) (125 mg Tiletamine & 125 mg Zolazepam)	Powder	250 mg	TiletamineZolazepam = 20 mg/ml (Tiletamine 10 mg/ml & Zolazepam 10 mg/ml)
Xylazine (20 mg/ml)	1.25 ml	25 mg	Xylazine = 2 mg/ml
Dist. water for Inj.	10 ml	....	....
Total	12.50 ml	....	....

The cost of the preparation would be approximately Rs. 127 per ml as per the MRP of each of the drugs.

Dose of BTDex/BTX for dogs and cats

For	Dose of BTDex/BTX	Route	Amount of drugs received per kg when administered at the specified volume		
			Butorphanol / Buprenorphine	Tiletamine-Zolazepam	Dexmed/ Xylazine
Mild to moderate sedation	0.05 ml/kg (0.5 ml/10 kg)	IM	Butorphanol @ 0.05 mg/kg / Buprenorphine @ 0.0015 mg/kg	1 mg/kg	Dex 2.5 mcg/kg or Xyl 0.1 mg/kg
Profound sedation	0.1 ml/kg 1) ml/10 kg)	IM	Butorphanol @ 0.1 mg/kg / Buprenorphine @ 0.003 mg/kg	2 mg/kg	Dex 5 mcg/kg or Xyl 0.2 mg/kg
Light surgical plane	0.15 ml/kg (1.5 ml/10 kg)	IM	Butorphanol @ 0.15 mg/kg / Buprenorphine @ 0.0045 mg/kg	3 mg/kg	Dex 7.5 mcg/kg or Xyl 0.3 mg/kg
Deep surgical plane	0.2 ml/kg (2 ml/10 kg)	IM	Butorphanol @ 0.2 mg/kg / Buprenorphine @ 0.006 mg/kg	4 mg/kg	Dex 10 mcg/kg or Xyl 0.4 mg/kg

The great flexibility in dose range (from 0.05 to 0.2 ml per kilogram IM), permits a practitioner to decide the dose rate based on the age of the animal, health status and type of surgery. Mild to moderate sedation can be achieved by intramuscular administration of 0.05 ml of the combination per kilogram body weight. Profound sedation could be achieved with intramuscular administration of 0.1 ml of the combination per kilogram body weight. Larger doses increase the depth of sedation to the level of light and deep planes of anaesthesia. With higher doses, animals very quickly attain recumbency and surgical plane of anaesthesia. The onset of action is rapid and lasts for more than 30 minutes. Duration of anaesthesia and duration of recovery increases with the dose. Also, the cardiorespiratory depression would be more profound with the larger doses. Animals other than healthy adults, should be administered smaller doses of the combination. The respiratory depression that happens should be managed by assisting the ventilation using enriched oxygen, for which the patients very well respond to. Respiratory depression usually subsides with surgical stimulation (Eger *et al*., 1972; Ko and Berman, 2010; Ko and Krimins, 2013).

References

Cagle, L. A., Franzi, L. M., Epstein, S. E., Kass, P. H., Last, J. A. and Kenyon, N. J. 2017. Injectable Anesthesia for Mice: Combined Effects of Dexmedetomidine, Tiletamine-Zolazepam, and Butorphanol. Anesth. Res. Pract. 17: 1–7.

Eger, E. I., Dolan, W. M., Stevens, W. C., Miller, R. D. and Way, W. L. 1972. Surgical Stimulation Antagonizes the Respiratory Depression Produced by Forane. Anesthesiology. 36(6): 544–549.

Ko, J. C., Krimins, R. A., Weil, A. B. and Payton, M. E. 2012. Evaluation of anesthetic, analgesic, and cardiorespiratory effects in dogs after intramuscular administration of dexmedetomidine–butorphanol–tiletamine-zolazepam or dexmedetomidine-tramadol-ketamine drug combinations. Am. J. Vet. Res. 73(11): 1707-1714.

Ko, J.C. 2013. Injectable Sedative and Anesthesia - Analgesia combinations in dogs and cats. In: Small animal anaesthesia and pain management - A color handbook, Mansion Publishing Ltd. pp. 199-223.

Ko, J.C. and Berman, A.G. 2010. Anesthesia in Shelter Medicine. Topics in companion Anim. Med. 25(2):92-97.

Ko, J.C. and Krimins, R.A. 2013. Anesthesia in shelter medicine and high volume/high quality spay and neuter programs. In: Small animal anaesthesia and pain management - A color handbook, 2nd Ed., Mansion Publishing Ltd. pp. 311-322.

Nesgash, A., Yaregal, B., Kindu, T. and Hailu, E. 2016. Evalution of General Anesthesia Using Xylazine-Ketamine Combination with and without Diazepam for Ovariohysterectomy in Bitches. J. Vet. Sci. Tech. 07(06): 1-6.

Sooryadas S., Verma, A., Souljai, J.S., Dinesh, P.T., Varghese, R. and Jineshkumar, N.S., 2019. Theory of multimodal balanced anaesthesia and its practice. J. Indian Vet. Assoc., 17(3): 7-11.

Verma, A., Sooryadas, S., Dinesh P.T. and Chandy, G. 2019. Dexmed-butorphanol-midazolam-Ketamine anaesthesia followed by Dexmed-Midazolam-Lignocaine-ketamine CRI. J. Indian Vet. Assoc., 17(3): 56-58.

Verma, A., Sooryadas, S., Dinesh P.T., Chandy, G. and Caulkett, N. 2020. Continuous rate infusion anaesthesia with dexmedetomidine-midazolam-ketamine-lignocaine in dogs. Indian. J. Vet. Surg. 41(2): 104-106.

5

Cocktails for Total Intravenous Anaesthesia (TIVA)

Total Intravenous Anaesthesia

Maintenance of anaesthesia, conventionally, is done either with inhalants, or as intermittent boli of injectable anaesthetics. The pharmacological complexity of the uptake and elimination of inhalant anaesthetic agents, and the need of technical and functional knowhow, of inhalant anaesthesia machine, either restricts its use in majority clinical practice, or is not used in an ideal manner. Injectable anaesthetic drugs as intermittent boli "as and when needed" is the practice by majority practitioners for maintenance of anaesthesia. Intermittent bolus injections of anaesthetic drugs creates intermittent peaks of anaesthesia and thereby increased side effects due to high doses. Instead, a continuous rate infusion of the anaesthetic drugs, in smaller quantities is employed in TIVA, providing balanced anaesthetic maintenance. These drugs act through different pathways, providing analgesia, muscle relaxation and unconsciousness, in a synergistic manner. TIVA is thus a technique in which anaesthesia is maintained solely through the use of intravenous drugs, without reliance on inhaled anaesthetics (Kennedy, 2016).

Total intravenous anaesthesia is commonly achieved using a combination of sedative-hypnotics, analgesics and even muscle relaxation drugs, often administered via continuous rate infusion (CRI) to maintain stable drug levels (Verma *et al.*, 2020). The key advantage of TIVA is that it provide stable haemodynamics because it maintains the sympathetic tone well. Also, this procedure promises less environmental contamination avoiding exposure to anaesthetic gas in the operating rooms. TIVA is emerging as a popular option in a range of surgical procedures due to its benefits in patient comfort, recovery, and control over anaesthesia depth.

Few examples of anaesthetic cocktails for total intravenous anaesthesia in dogs through constant rate infusion are mentioned below. Easy understanding on how to calculate and prepare CRI is mentioned later.

1. Dexmedetomidine (2 mcg/kg/hr), midazolam (3 mcg/kg/min), lignocaine (50 mcg/kg/min) and ketamine (40 mcg/kg/min) as a cocktail intravenous infusion in normal saline. Anaesthesia is induced by intramuscular administration of a cocktail of DBMK mentioned in earlier chapter, followed by an intravenous loading dose of lignocaine at the rate of 2 mg/kg prior to the cocktail intravenous infusion (Verma *et al.*, 2020).
2. Xylazine (1 mg/kg/hr), midazolam (3 mcg/kg/min), lignocaine (50 mcg/kg/min) and ketamine (40 mcg/kg/min) as a cocktail intravenous infusion in

normal saline. Anaesthesia is induced by intramuscular administration of a cocktail of xylazine (0.4 mg/kg), butorphanol (0.2 mg/kg), midazolam (0.2 mg/kg) and ketamine (10 mg/kg), followed by an intravenous loading dose of lignocaine at the rate of 2 mg/kg prior to the cocktail intravenous infusion (Kenjale, 2022).

3. Dexmedetomidine (2 mcg/kg/hr), lignocaine (50 mcg/kg/min) and ketamine (40 mcg/kg/min) as a cocktail intravenous infusion in normal saline, alongside another intravenous infusion of propofol (50 mcg/kg/min) in normal saline through a 3-way stopcock. General anaesthesia is induced as follows - sedation using a combination of tiletamine-zolazepam (2 mg/kg) – butorphanol (0.2 mg/kg) – dexmedetomidine (5 mcg/kg) in a single syringe administered intramuscularly followed by induction with diluted propofol administered intravenous "to effect". Following induction of anaesthesia, an intravenous loading dose of lignocaine (2 mg/kg IV) is administered prior to the cocktail intravenous infusion (Chandramohan *et al.*, 2024).

The protocols provide very good to excellent intra-operative analgesia, muscle relaxation and unconsciousness (Liptak, 2022; Verma *et al.* 2020; Kenjale *et al.*, 2022 and Chandramohan *et al.*, 2024). Reduction in heart rate and pulse rate should be expected due to the alpha 2 adrenoceptor agonist in the cocktails, but the mean arterial blood pressure would be maintained, ensuring adequate organ and tissue perfusion, evident from normal capillary refill times. Respiratory depression and reduction in ventilation should be expected following induction, till commencement of the surgical stimulation. When found so, the breaths of the patient should be assisted by gently squeezing the reservoir/rebreathing bag to maintain eucapnia, till the sympathetic stimulation out of surgical manoeuvres improves ventilatory drives. Nociception if noticed with very severe painful orthopaedic manoeuvres shall be managed by supplementing intravenous ketamine or fentanyl at its analgesic doses.

Preparation of Constant Rate Infusions for TIVA

Constant/continuous rate infusion (CRI) helps administer drugs at a consistent rate instead of giving them as bolus injections. Various intravenous analgesic/sedative/muscle relaxant/anaesthetic drugs which are pharmacologically and chemically compatible can be used at minimal doses as a cocktail for the CRI. The CRI ensures a steady flow of the drug(s) maintaining the required plasma concentration of the drug(s) to sustain analgesia, sedation, muscle relaxation and/or unconsciousness throughout the procedure, reducing/avoiding the requirement of gaseous agents for maintenance of anaesthesia.

Due to the complexity of mathematical calculations, many of us are hesitant to use CRIs on our daily practice. Once we integrate CRIs into our anaesthetic / pain management routines, we truly start appreciating the effectiveness and elegance of this technique in maintaining the triads of anaesthesia.

There are many ready-to-use worksheets and mobile/online applications used to calculate CRI drug volumes and infusions. Understanding their basics will help anyone do it without depending on any formulas/worksheets or online applications. The steps below help a better understanding for calculating and preparing CRIs.

Basic understanding of CRI calculation

First ask yourself the following two questions –

1. At what CRI dose [mg (or mcg)/kg/hr] the drug has to be administered?
   ....**A** [mg (or mcg)/kg/hr]
2. At what fluid rate (ml/kg/hr) you will be administering the drug infusion?
   ....**B** (ml/kg/hr)

   From the above two answers, understand that you need to prepare **A** mg (or mcg) of your drug in every **B** ml of infusion fluid. When this infusion is administered at a rate of **B** ml/kg/hr, it will deliver the drug at a constant rate infusion (CRI) dose of **A** mg (or mcg)/kg/hr.

   Let us see how this infusion has to be made.
3. Divide **A** with **B**.

   This gives you the concentration of your drug per every milliliter [mg (or mcg) of drug per ml] of your infusion .... **X** [**A** mg (or mcg) per **B** ml]
4. Now ask yourself what is the fluid infusion (normal saline) bag/bottle (100 ml/500 ml/1000 ml) that you will use for preparing/delivering the CRI? ......**C** (ml)
5. Multiply **X** (**A** mg/mcg per **B** ml) with **C** (ml).......... **Y** [mg (or mcg)]

   This is the total quantity [mg (or mcg)] of your drug which is required to prepare the infusion in that fluid infusion **C**.
6. Divide **Y** with the presentation of the drug. This gives you the volume of the drug required to prepare the CRI .... **Z** (ml)
7. Withdraw and discard **Z** ml from the normal saline fluid bag and then add **Z** ml of your drug to prepare the CRI.

Administer the above infusion at **B** ml/kg/hr to deliver your drug at the CRI dose of **A** mg (or mcg) per kg/hr.

Examples

1. Lignocaine (20 mg/ml presentation) has to be delivered as CRI @ 50 mcg/kg/min intra-operatively; fluid rate = 10 ml/kg/hr; fluid infusion volume (fluid bag to which CRI is to be made) = 500 ml

CRI dose of lignocaine	= 50 mcg/kg/min
	= 50 mcg/kg/min x 60 min/hr
	= 3000 mcg/kg/hr
	= 3 mg/kg/hr ....**A**
Fluid rate	= 10 ml/kg/hr .... **B**
Total infusion fluid volume	= 500 ml ....**C**

- From the above, it is understood that there should be 3 mg of lignocaine in every 10 ml of your infusion.
- i.e. 0.3 mg of lignocaine in every ml of infusion.
- If it is so, then 500 ml of infusion should have 0.3 mg x 500 = 150 mg lignocaine.
- So you need 150 mg of lignocaine to prepare the infusion.
- i.e. 7.5 ml of lignocaine (Lignocaine is available as 20 mg/ml presentation)

Knowing 7.5 ml lignocaine is needed for preparing the CRI, first withdraw and discard 7.5 ml of normal saline from the 500 ml fluid bag/bottle; then add your 7.5 ml lignocaine into the bag of normal saline to prepare the CRI infusion. This infusion when delivered at 10 ml/kg/hr provides lignocaine at the CRI dose of 3 mg/kg/hr (50 mcg/kg/min). A loading dose of lignocaine @ 2 mg/kg should be administered intravenously before starting the CRI. The loading dose of the drug will help achieve its target drug level in the plasma which is then maintained by the CRI.

Steps involved for calculation

Divide **A** with **B** (to know the concentration of lignocaine in unit volume of the infusion)	= 3 mg lignocaine / 10 ml infusion **X**
Multiply **X** with **C** = (to know the total amount of lignocaine needed to prepare the infusion)	$\frac{\text{3 mg lignocaine}}{\text{10 ml infusion}}$ x 500 ml infusion = 150 mg lignocaine .....**Y**
Divide **Y** with the presentation of lignocaine (to get the volume of lignocaine needed to prepare the CRI infusion)	= $\frac{\text{150 mg lignocaine}}{\text{20 mg/ml}}$ = 7.5 ml lignocaine

2. Dexmedetomidine (@ 2 mcg/kg/hr), lignocaine (@ 50 mcg/kg/min) and ketamine (@ 40 mcg/kg/min) has to be administered intra-operatively as a cocktail intravenous infusion in 500 ml normal saline at a fluid rate of 5 ml/kg/hr, alongside another intravenous infusion of propofol (@ 50 mcg/kg/min) in 500 ml normal saline at a fluid rate of 5 ml/kg/hr.

   CRI Infusion No. 1 – DLK Infusion

   CRI dose of Dexmedetomidine = 2 mcg/kg/hr

   CRI dose of Lignocaine = 50 mcg/kg/min = 3 mg/kg/hr

   CRI dose of Ketamine = 40 mcg/kg/min = 2.4 mg/kg/hr

   Fluid rate and Volume of normal saline for preparing CRI = 5 ml/kg/hr; 500 ml

   From the figures mentioned above, it should be understood that if there is 2 mcg of dexmedetomidine, 3 mg of lignocaine and 2.4 mg of ketamine each in 5 ml of the fluid, and administering that fluid infusion at 5 ml/kg/hr will deliver the dexmedetomidine, lignocaine and ketamine at the respective CRI doses mentioned above.

The volume of the above drugs needed for preparing CRI can then be calculated as follows:

For Dexmedetomidine $= \frac{2 \text{ mcg dexmedetomidine x } 500 \text{ ml}}{5 \text{ ml}}$

$= 200$ mcg

$= \frac{200 \text{ mcg}}{100 \text{ mcg/ml}}$

$= 2$ ml of dexmedetomidine (presentation 100 mcg/ml)

For Lignocaine $= \frac{3 \text{ mg lignocaine x } 500 \text{ ml}}{5 \text{ ml}}$

$= 300$ mg

$= \frac{300 \text{ mg}}{20 \text{ mg/ml}}$

$= 15$ ml of lignocaine (presentation 20 mg/ml)

For Ketamine $= \frac{2.4 \text{ mg ketamine}}{5 \text{ ml}} \text{ x } 500 \text{ ml}$

$= 240$ mg

$= \frac{240 \text{ mg}}{50 \text{ mg/ml}}$

$= 4.8$ ml of ketamine (presentation 50 mg/ml)

Total volume of the above drugs = 2 + 15 + 4.8 = 21.8 ml

To prepare the CRI infusion of DLK, withdraw and discard 21.8 ml of normal saline from the fluid bag. Then add the above 21.8 ml of the drugs to make it up to 500 ml infusion. Administering this infusion at the rate of 5 ml/kg/hr will deliver the drugs at their respective CRI doses.

CRI Infusion No. 2 – Propofol Infusion

Propofol infusion can also be prepared as detailed above, and administered at the rate of 5 ml/kg/hr which will deliver propofol @ 50 mcg/kg/min.

The infusions 1 and 2 can then be administered simultaneously through a three-way stopcock using a volumetric infusion pump.

References

Chandramohan S., Sooryadas S., Dinesh P.T., Jineshkumar N.S., Remya V., Anoop S. and David P.V. (2024). Multimodal balanced general anaesthesia using tiletamine-zolazepam, butorphanol, dexmedetomidine, propofol, ketamine and lignocaine in dogs. Indian J. Vet. Surg. 45(1):21-26

Dugdale A.H.A., Beaumont G., Bradbrook C. and Gurney M. (2020). Analgesic infusions In: Veterinary Anaesthesia Principles to Practice. (2nd ed.). Wiley Blackwell. pp. 95-97

Kenjale L., Varghese R., Dinesh P.T., Sooryadas S. and Umesh C.G. (2022). Evaluation of xylazine-midazolam-lignocaine-ketamine constant rate infusion (CRI) for maintenance in xylazine-butorphanol-midazolam-ketamine (XBMK) anaesthetised dogs. JIVA. 20(2):51-59

Kennedy, M.J. 2016. Total Intravenous Anaesthesia (TIVA) In: Questions and answers in small animal anaesthesia (1st ed.). Smith L.J. (Ed.). John Wiley & Sons. pp.101-105

Kerr C. (2016). Constant Rate Infusions In: Questions and answers in small animal anaesthesia (1st ed.). Smith L.J. (Ed.). John Wiley & Sons. pp.163-171

Ko J.C. (2013). Acute pain management In: Anaesthesia and pain management in dogs and cats – A colour handbook (1st ed.). Mansion Publishing Ltd. pp. 284-287

Lakshmi S.S.S., Sooryadas S., Jineshkumar N.S., Sudhir P.H., Anoop S., Remya V. and Dinesh P.T. (2024). Clinical efficacy of procedural sedation combined with femoral and sciatic nerve blocks for stifle and tibial surgeries in dogs. Indian J. Vet. Surg. 45(1):14-20

Liptak T., Kuricova M. and Capik I. (2012). Use of total intravenous anaesthesia (TIVA) in dogs – A review. Folia Veterinaria 56(4):39-47

McKiernan E.P. (1985). An even simpler way to determine drug infusion rates. Anaesthesiology 63:459

Verma A., Sooryadas S., Dinesh P.T., Chandy G. and Caulkett N. (2020). Continuous rate infusion anaesthesia with dexmedetomidine-midazolam-ketamine-lignocaine in dogs. Indian J. Vet. Surg. 41(2):104-106

Index

About the Author

Dr. Sooryadas graduated in 1998 from the College of Veterinary & Animal Sciences, Mannuthy, Kerala. He completed his Masters in Veterinary Surgery & Radiology (1998-2000) from the same college with anaesthesia as his research topic, and his PhD in Veterinary Surgery at Madras Veterinary College (2007-2010), specializing in ophthalmology. Dr. Sooryadas has served in the Kerala State Animal Husbandry Department, worked as faculty at Kerala Veterinary & Animal Sciences University, and was a guide for Masters and Doctoral scholars in their research works on anaesthesiology and ophthalmology, and Post-Graduate Diploma students in anaesthesiology. He regularly offers hands-on trainings for practitioners in veterinary anaesthesiology and ophthalmology. He has authored numerous publications in national and international journals and received many awards and honours. Dr. Sooryadas has been invited internationally, including to the Republic of Seychelles for establishing inhalant anaesthesia facilities and conducting ophthalmology camp, in recognition to which he had been honoured by the University for extending the clinical expertise of the University to another country. Notably, during the COVID-19 lockdown, he successfully tele-guided anaesthesia and surgery for rare surgical conditions – persistent right aortic arch, patent ductus arteriosum and cricopharyngeal achalasia in small puppies stationed in Malaysia, marking a milestone in veterinary medicine in India. He is skilled in laparoscopic surgery, soft tissue surgeries, orthopaedics, and anaesthesiology. He was the Head of the Department of Veterinary Surgery and Radiology at College of Veterinary and Animal Sciences, Kerala Veterinary and Animal Sciences Unviersity, Pookode, Wayanad. Taking few years' leave from the University, he is currently working as the Chief Surgeon at Charis Veterinary Clinic in Bahrain, and Professor and Program Director for Charis Vets Educational.

Contributors

Dinesh P.T., MVSc, PhD.
Associate Professor and Head
Department of Veterinary Surgery & Radiology
College of Veterinary & Animal Sciences, Pookode
Kerala Veterinary & Animal Sciences University, Pookode, Wayanad, Kerala

Jineshkumar N.S., MVSc
Assistant Professor
Department of Veterinary Surgery & Radiology
College of Veterinary & Animal Sciences, Pookode
Kerala Veterinary & Animal Sciences University, Pookode, Wayanad, Kerala

Remya V., MVSc, PhD.
Assistant Professor
Department of Veterinary Surgery & Radiology
College of Veterinary & Animal Sciences, Kerala Veterinary & Animal Sciences University, Pookode, Wayanad, Kerala